DR. BARBARA'S 7 DAYS FULL-BODY DETOx

The simple guide to harnessing the power of juice recipes, smoothies and diets for optimal and cleanse of your kidney, liver, lungs, skin, and whole body

Mauricio Andrea

Table of Contents

COPYRIGHT © 2023

CHAPTER ONE

Introduction to Dr. Barbara's Herbal 7-Day Full Body Detox

Detoxification has been a subject of interest for millennia, with cultures worldwide embracing various methods to cleanse the body and rejuvenate health. In contemporary times, as lifestyles become increasingly hectic and diets more processed, the need for detoxification has gained prominence. Among the myriad of detox programs available, Dr. Barbara's Herbal 7-Day Full Body Detox stands out as a comprehensive and holistic approach to purifying the body.

Understanding Detoxification

Before delving into the specifics of Dr. Barbara's program, it's crucial to understand the concept of detoxification. Detoxification refers to the process of eliminating toxins and impurities from the body, primarily through the liver, kidneys, skin, lungs, and lymphatic system. These toxins can originate from various sources, including environmental pollutants, processed foods, medications, and metabolic waste products.

Over time, the body's natural detoxification pathways may become overwhelmed, leading to a buildup of toxins, which can contribute to fatigue, digestive issues, inflammation, and a weakened immune system. Detox programs aim to support the body's natural detoxification processes, allowing it to efficiently eliminate accumulated toxins and restore optimal functioning.

The Importance of Herbal Remedies

Herbal remedies have been utilized for centuries across cultures worldwide for their therapeutic properties. Unlike synthetic drugs, which often come with side effects and long-term risks, herbal remedies offer a natural and gentle approach to promoting health and well-being. Many herbs possess detoxifying properties, supporting the body's organs in the elimination of toxins while nourishing and replenishing vital nutrients.

Dr. Barbara's Herbal 7-Day Full Body Detox harnesses the power of carefully selected herbs known for their detoxifying, antioxidant, and anti-inflammatory properties. These herbs work synergistically to cleanse the body from within, targeting specific organs and systems involved in the detoxification process.

The Science Behind Dr. Barbara's Formula

Dr. Barbara's Herbal 7-Day Full Body Detox is backed by scientific research and formulated based on principles of herbal medicine, nutrition, and detoxification. Each herb included in the program is chosen for its unique therapeutic benefits and compatibility with the body's natural detox pathways.

For example, ingredients such as dandelion root and milk thistle are renowned for their liver-supporting properties, helping to enhance liver function and bile production, crucial for the elimination of toxins. Burdock root and red clover assist in purifying the blood and lymphatic system, while psyllium husk and slippery elm bark promote digestive health and regularity, facilitating the removal of waste and toxins from the colon.

The Comprehensive Approach

What sets Dr. Barbara's Herbal 7-Day Full Body Detox apart is its comprehensive approach to detoxification. Rather than focusing solely on one aspect of detoxification, such as fasting or juice cleanses, this program addresses multiple facets of the body's detox pathways, ensuring a thorough and effective cleanse.

The program consists of a carefully curated combination of herbal supplements, dietary recommendations, hydration protocols, and lifestyle modifications designed to support detoxification at every level. By incorporating these elements synergistically, Dr. Barbara's program maximizes the body's ability to eliminate toxins while minimizing detox symptoms and promoting overall well-being.

The Seven-Day Protocol

Dr. Barbara's Herbal 7-Day Full Body Detox is designed to be completed over a seven-day period, providing a structured yet flexible approach to detoxification. Each day of the program is meticulously planned to optimize detox outcomes while accommodating individual preferences and lifestyles.

The protocol typically begins with a preparation phase, during which participants gradually transition to a clean, whole foods-based diet and begin taking herbal supplements to prime the body for detoxification. Throughout the seven days, participants adhere to a specific regimen of herbal supplements, dietary guidelines, and hydration protocols, with ample support and guidance provided along the way.

Benefits of Dr. Barbara's Herbal 7-Day Full Body Detox

The benefits of completing Dr. Barbara's Herbal 7-Day Full Body Detox extend far beyond mere detoxification. While the primary goal is to rid the body of accumulated toxins, participants often report experiencing a myriad of additional benefits, including increased energy levels, improved digestion, clearer skin, better sleep quality, and enhanced mental clarity.

By supporting the body's natural detoxification processes and promoting overall health and vitality, Dr. Barbara's program empowers individuals to take control of their well-being and embark on a path to long-term health and wellness.

Conclusion

In conclusion, Dr. Barbara's Herbal 7-Day Full Body Detox offers a comprehensive and scientifically backed approach to detoxification, harnessing the power of herbal remedies to support the body's natural detox pathways. By addressing multiple facets of detoxification and providing structured guidance and support, this program enables individuals to cleanse their bodies effectively while promoting overall health and vitality. Whether you're looking to jumpstart a healthier lifestyle, overcome fatigue and digestive issues, or simply rejuvenate your health, Dr. Barbara's Herbal 7-Day Full Body Detox provides a safe, effective, and transformative solution.

CHAPTER TWO

Understanding the Importance of Detoxification for Health

Detoxification, often shortened to "detox," has become a buzzword in health and wellness circles, but its significance goes far beyond trendy diets or fleeting fads. At its core, detoxification is a fundamental process vital for maintaining optimal health and well-being. In this comprehensive exploration, we'll delve into the importance of detoxification for health, examining its role in the body, the benefits it offers, and strategies for supporting natural detoxification pathways.

The Body's Natural Detoxification Pathways

Detoxification is a complex physiological process orchestrated by the body's organs and systems to eliminate harmful substances and waste products. The primary organs involved in detoxification include the liver, kidneys, skin, lungs, and lymphatic system.

1. **Liver:** Often referred to as the body's detox powerhouse, the liver plays a central role in detoxification by metabolizing and neutralizing toxins. It transforms harmful substances into water-soluble compounds that can be excreted via bile or urine.

2. **Kidneys:** The kidneys filter waste products and toxins from the bloodstream, regulating fluid balance and electrolyte

levels. They excrete waste in the form of urine, helping to maintain internal equilibrium.

3. **Skin:** As the body's largest organ, the skin serves as a vital detoxification pathway through sweat production. Sweating allows for the elimination of toxins, heavy metals, and metabolic waste products, supporting overall detoxification.

4. **Lungs:** The lungs play a role in detoxification by expelling volatile organic compounds and other airborne toxins through respiration. Deep breathing techniques can enhance lung detoxification and oxygenate the body.

5. **Lymphatic System:** Often referred to as the body's drainage system, the lymphatic system helps remove toxins and waste from tissues and transport them to lymph nodes for filtration and elimination.

The Impact of Toxins on Health

In today's modern world, we are exposed to a myriad of toxins and pollutants on a daily basis. These toxins can originate from various sources, including air pollution, contaminated water, processed foods, household chemicals, medications, and personal care products. Prolonged exposure to toxins can overwhelm the body's detoxification pathways, leading to a buildup of toxins in tissues and organs.

The accumulation of toxins can have far-reaching effects on health, contributing to a wide range of symptoms and chronic conditions, including:

1. **Fatigue:** Toxins interfere with cellular energy production and mitochondrial function, leading to fatigue and low energy levels.

2. **Digestive Issues:** Toxins can disrupt gut microbiota balance, impair digestion, and contribute to symptoms such as bloating, constipation, and food sensitivities.

3. **Inflammation:** Chronic exposure to toxins can trigger inflammatory responses in the body, contributing to inflammation-related conditions such as arthritis, autoimmune diseases, and cardiovascular disease.

4. **Immune Dysfunction:** Toxins compromise immune function by overloading the body's detoxification pathways and triggering immune system dysregulation, increasing susceptibility to infections and chronic illnesses.

5. **Neurological Symptoms:** Some toxins have neurotoxic effects, affecting brain function and cognitive health, leading to symptoms such as brain fog, memory impairment, and mood disorders.

The Benefits of Detoxification

Engaging in regular detoxification practices can yield numerous benefits for overall health and well-being. By supporting the body's natural detoxification pathways, individuals may experience:

1. **Increased Energy and Vitality:** Detoxification helps remove metabolic waste products and toxins that can drain energy levels, leading to increased vitality and improved stamina.

2. **Improved Digestion:** Cleansing the digestive system can promote optimal gut health, enhance nutrient absorption, and alleviate symptoms of bloating, gas, and indigestion.

3. **Enhanced Immune Function:** Supporting detoxification pathways strengthens the immune system, reducing the burden of toxins and pathogens and enhancing the body's ability to fight infections.

4. **Clearer Skin:** Detoxification can improve skin health by reducing inflammation, eliminating toxins that contribute to acne and other skin conditions, and promoting a radiant complexion.

5. **Mental Clarity and Focus:** Removing toxins from the body can sharpen cognitive function, improve mental clarity, and enhance focus and concentration.

6. **Weight Management:** Detoxification can support weight loss efforts by optimizing metabolic function, balancing hormones, and reducing cravings for processed foods and sugar.

Strategies for Supporting Detoxification

While the body has innate detoxification mechanisms, supporting these processes through lifestyle practices and dietary choices can optimize detoxification and promote overall health. Some strategies for supporting detoxification include:

1. **Eat a Nutrient-Dense Diet:** Focus on whole, unprocessed foods rich in vitamins, minerals, antioxidants, and fiber to support detoxification pathways and nourish the body.

2. **Stay Hydrated:** Drink plenty of water to support kidney function and promote the elimination of toxins through urine.

3. **Exercise Regularly:** Engage in regular physical activity to stimulate circulation, lymphatic drainage, and sweat production, supporting detoxification and overall health.

4. **Practice Stress Management:** Chronic stress can impair detoxification pathways and compromise immune function. Incorporate stress-reducing practices such as meditation, yoga, deep breathing exercises, and adequate sleep to support detoxification and overall well-being.

5. **Limit Exposure to Toxins:** Minimize exposure to environmental toxins by choosing organic foods, using natural household cleaning and personal care products, and avoiding tobacco smoke, air pollution, and excessive alcohol consumption.

6. **Consider Detox Protocols:** Periodic detox protocols, such as juice cleanses, herbal detox programs, or intermittent fasting, can provide additional support for detoxification and promote overall health and vitality.

Conclusion

In conclusion, detoxification plays a pivotal role in maintaining optimal health and well-being by eliminating toxins and waste products from the body. By supporting the body's natural detoxification pathways through lifestyle practices, dietary choices, and periodic detox protocols, individuals can experience increased energy, improved digestion, enhanced immune function, clearer skin, and mental clarity. Prioritizing detoxification as part of a holistic approach to health can empower individuals to thrive and live vibrant, fulfilling lives.

CHAPTER THREE

Dr. Barbara's Holistic Approach to Full Body Detoxification

Dr. Barbara's holistic approach to full body detoxification embodies a comprehensive and integrative methodology aimed at promoting wellness on multiple levels. Unlike traditional detox programs that may focus solely on one aspect of cleansing, such as dietary modifications or herbal supplements, Dr. Barbara's approach encompasses a wide array of modalities designed to support the body's natural detoxification pathways while nurturing overall health and vitality. In this exploration, we'll delve into the key components of Dr. Barbara's holistic approach and how they work synergistically to facilitate full body detoxification.

1. Herbal Supplementation:

At the core of Dr. Barbara's approach are carefully selected herbal supplements formulated to target specific organs and systems involved in detoxification. These supplements are crafted from high-quality botanical ingredients known for their detoxifying, antioxidant, and anti-inflammatory properties. Each herb is chosen for its unique therapeutic benefits and compatibility with the body's natural detox pathways.

For example, ingredients like dandelion root and milk thistle support liver function, aiding in the metabolism and elimination of toxins. Burdock root and red clover assist in purifying the blood and lymphatic system, while psyllium husk and slippery elm bark promote digestive health and regularity, facilitating the removal of waste and toxins from the colon.

2. Nutritional Guidance:

In addition to herbal supplementation, Dr. Barbara's holistic approach includes dietary recommendations aimed at supporting detoxification and nourishing the body with essential nutrients. Participants are encouraged to consume a clean, whole foods-based diet rich in fruits, vegetables, lean proteins, healthy fats, and fiber. By emphasizing nutrient-dense foods and minimizing processed and inflammatory foods, such as sugar, refined carbohydrates, and artificial additives, participants can optimize detoxification and promote overall health.

3. Hydration Protocols:

Proper hydration is essential for effective detoxification, as water plays a critical role in flushing toxins from the body via urine, sweat, and respiration. Dr. Barbara's approach includes hydration protocols designed to ensure adequate water intake throughout the detoxification process. Participants are encouraged to drink plenty of water, herbal teas, and hydrating fluids to support kidney function and promote the elimination of toxins.

4. Lifestyle Modifications:

In addition to herbal supplementation, dietary guidance, and hydration protocols, Dr. Barbara's holistic approach incorporates lifestyle modifications aimed at reducing toxin exposure and supporting overall well-being. Participants are encouraged to prioritize stress management techniques, such as meditation, yoga, deep breathing exercises, and adequate sleep, to promote relaxation and optimize detoxification.

Regular physical activity is also emphasized to stimulate circulation, lymphatic drainage, and sweat production, facilitating the elimination of toxins from the body. Participants are encouraged to engage in activities they enjoy, such as walking, jogging, cycling, or yoga, to promote movement and support detoxification.

5. Mind-Body Connection:

Dr. Barbara's holistic approach recognizes the interconnectedness of the mind and body and the profound impact that mental and emotional well-being can have on overall health. Participants are encouraged to cultivate mindfulness practices, such as meditation, journaling, or gratitude exercises, to foster a positive mindset and reduce stress levels.

By addressing the mind-body connection, Dr. Barbara's approach promotes holistic healing and empowers individuals to take an active role in their health and well-being. By nurturing the body, mind, and spirit, participants can achieve comprehensive detoxification and experience enhanced vitality, clarity, and resilience.

Conclusion:

In conclusion, Dr. Barbara's holistic approach to full body detoxification offers a comprehensive and integrative methodology for promoting wellness on multiple levels. By combining herbal supplementation, nutritional guidance, hydration protocols, lifestyle modifications, and mindfulness practices, Dr. Barbara's approach addresses detoxification from a holistic perspective, supporting the body's natural detox pathways while nurturing overall health and vitality. By embracing this holistic approach, individuals can achieve comprehensive detoxification and experience lasting benefits for their physical, mental, and emotional well-being.

CHAPTER FOUR

The Science Behind Detoxification: How Herbs Support Cleansing

Detoxification is a complex physiological process orchestrated by the body's organs and systems to eliminate harmful substances and waste products. While the body has innate detoxification mechanisms, various factors, including environmental toxins, poor diet, stress, and lifestyle habits, can overwhelm these pathways, leading to a buildup of toxins and metabolic waste. Herbs have long been utilized for their therapeutic properties, including their ability to support detoxification and promote overall health. In this exploration, we'll delve into the science behind detoxification and how herbs support cleansing processes.

1. Liver Support:

The liver plays a central role in detoxification, metabolizing and neutralizing toxins before they can be eliminated from the body. Several herbs have been shown to support liver function and enhance detoxification processes:

- **Milk Thistle (Silybum marianum):** One of the most well-known herbs for liver support, milk thistle contains a compound called silymarin, which has antioxidant and anti-inflammatory properties. Silymarin helps protect liver cells from damage caused by toxins and promotes regeneration of liver tissue.

- **Dandelion Root (Taraxacum officinale):** Dandelion root is rich in vitamins, minerals, and phytonutrients that support liver health. It stimulates bile production, which aids in the digestion and elimination of fats and toxins from the liver.

- **Turmeric (Curcuma longa):** Curcumin, the active compound in turmeric, exhibits potent antioxidant and anti-inflammatory properties. It helps protect the liver from damage caused by toxins and promotes the production of enzymes involved in detoxification.

2. Kidney Support:

The kidneys play a crucial role in filtering waste products and toxins from the bloodstream, regulating fluid balance, and maintaining electrolyte levels. Several herbs support kidney function and promote detoxification:

- **Nettle Leaf (Urtica dioica):** Nettle leaf is a diuretic herb that promotes urine production and helps flush out toxins from the kidneys. It also contains antioxidants that protect kidney cells from damage.

- **Dandelion Leaf (Taraxacum officinale):** In addition to its liver-supporting properties, dandelion leaf also acts as a diuretic, promoting kidney function and increasing urine output to facilitate toxin elimination.

- **Parsley (Petroselinum crispum):** Parsley is rich in antioxidants, vitamins, and minerals that support kidney health. It helps stimulate urine production and aids in the elimination of toxins and waste products.

3. Blood Purification:

Blood purification is essential for removing toxins and metabolic waste products from circulation and promoting overall health. Certain herbs possess blood-purifying properties and support detoxification:

- **Burdock Root (Arctium lappa):** Burdock root contains compounds called lignans, which have been shown to have blood-purifying effects. It supports liver function, enhances toxin elimination, and promotes clear, radiant skin.

- **Red Clover (Trifolium pratense):** Red clover is rich in antioxidants and phytochemicals that support blood purification and detoxification. It helps remove toxins from the bloodstream and supports lymphatic drainage.

- **Oregon Grape Root (Mahonia aquifolium):** Oregon grape root contains berberine, a compound with antimicrobial and blood-purifying properties. It supports liver function, enhances bile production, and aids in the elimination of toxins from the blood.

4. Digestive Support:

The digestive system plays a vital role in detoxification, as it is responsible for processing and eliminating toxins and waste products from the body. Several herbs support digestive health and promote detoxification:

- **Ginger (Zingiber officinale):** Ginger is a digestive tonic that helps stimulate digestion, reduce inflammation, and relieve gastrointestinal discomfort. It promotes detoxification by enhancing nutrient absorption and supporting regular bowel movements.

- **Peppermint (Mentha piperita):** Peppermint soothes digestive discomfort, reduces bloating and gas, and promotes healthy digestion. It supports detoxification by promoting bile flow and aiding in the elimination of toxins from the digestive tract.

- **Fennel (Foeniculum vulgare):** Fennel seeds contain compounds that support digestion and relieve gastrointestinal symptoms such as bloating, indigestion, and constipation. They help promote detoxification by supporting liver function and enhancing bile production.

Conclusion:

In conclusion, herbs play a crucial role in supporting detoxification processes by supporting the liver, kidneys, blood, and digestive system. Their therapeutic properties, including antioxidant, anti-inflammatory, diuretic, and blood-purifying effects, help enhance the body's natural detoxification pathways and promote overall health and well-being. Incorporating herbs into a balanced diet and lifestyle can support detoxification and contribute to optimal health and vitality.

CHAPTER FIVE

Essential Herbs for Detoxifying the Body and Boosting Vitality

Herbs have been valued for centuries for their therapeutic properties, including their ability to support detoxification and promote overall vitality. Incorporating these essential herbs into your daily routine can help cleanse the body of toxins, support organ function, and enhance overall well-being. In this exploration, we'll highlight some key herbs renowned for their detoxifying properties and their contributions to boosting vitality.

1. Milk Thistle (Silybum marianum):

Milk thistle is perhaps one of the most well-known herbs for liver support and detoxification. It contains a compound called silymarin, which has potent antioxidant and anti-inflammatory properties. Silymarin helps protect liver cells from damage caused by toxins, promotes regeneration of liver tissue, and enhances the liver's ability to metabolize and eliminate toxins from the body. Incorporating milk thistle into your routine can support overall liver health and promote detoxification.

2. Dandelion Root (Taraxacum officinale):

Dandelion root is another powerful herb renowned for its detoxifying properties. It stimulates bile production and flow, which aids in the digestion and elimination of fats and toxins from the liver. Dandelion root also acts as a diuretic, promoting kidney function and increasing urine output to facilitate toxin elimination. Additionally, dandelion root contains antioxidants that help protect liver cells from damage and support overall detoxification and vitality.

3. Burdock Root (Arctium lappa):

Burdock root is rich in antioxidants and compounds called lignans, which have blood-purifying effects. It supports liver function, enhances toxin elimination, and promotes clear, radiant skin. Burdock root also contains prebiotic fibers that nourish beneficial gut bacteria and support digestive health. By supporting liver function and promoting detoxification, burdock root contributes to overall vitality and well-being.

4. Turmeric (Curcuma longa):

Turmeric is a golden-yellow spice renowned for its anti-inflammatory and antioxidant properties. Its active compound, curcumin, helps protect the liver from damage caused by toxins, reduce inflammation, and promote bile production. Turmeric also supports digestive health by stimulating digestion, reducing bloating and gas, and supporting liver function. Incorporating turmeric into your diet or taking a curcumin supplement can support detoxification and boost vitality.

5. Ginger (Zingiber officinale):

Ginger is a warming herb that has been used for centuries to support digestion, reduce inflammation, and promote detoxification. It stimulates digestion, relieves gastrointestinal discomfort, and supports liver function. Ginger also has antioxidant and anti-inflammatory properties that help protect cells from damage and promote overall vitality. Enjoying ginger tea or adding fresh ginger to your meals can support detoxification and enhance well-being.

6. Nettle Leaf (Urtica dioica):

Nettle leaf is a nutrient-rich herb that supports detoxification and promotes overall vitality. It acts as a diuretic, promoting urine production and helping flush out toxins from the kidneys. Nettle leaf is also rich in vitamins, minerals, and antioxidants that support kidney function and protect against oxidative stress. Incorporating nettle leaf into your diet or enjoying nettle tea can support detoxification and boost vitality.

7. Red Clover (Trifolium pratense):

Red clover is a blood-purifying herb that supports detoxification and promotes overall health. It helps remove toxins from the bloodstream, supports lymphatic drainage, and promotes clear, radiant skin. Red clover is also rich in antioxidants and phytochemicals that support liver function and protect against cellular damage. Incorporating red clover into your routine can support detoxification and enhance vitality.

Conclusion:

In conclusion, incorporating essential herbs like milk thistle, dandelion root, burdock root, turmeric, ginger, nettle leaf, and red clover into your daily routine can support detoxification and promote overall vitality. These herbs support liver function, enhance toxin elimination, and protect against oxidative stress, helping cleanse the body of toxins and boost overall well-being. Whether enjoyed as teas, tinctures, or supplements, these herbs can be valuable allies in supporting your body's natural detoxification processes and enhancing vitality.

CHAPTER SIX

Dr. Barbara's Herbal Detox Protocol for the 7-Day Program

Dr. Barbara's Herbal Detox Protocol offers a structured and comprehensive approach to cleansing the body and rejuvenating health over a seven-day period. This program is designed to support the body's natural detoxification pathways, promote optimal organ function, and enhance overall vitality. In this detailed guide, we'll outline Dr. Barbara's Herbal Detox Protocol, including herbal supplements, dietary recommendations, hydration protocols, and lifestyle modifications for each day of the program.

Day 1: Preparation Phase

- **Herbal Supplements:** Begin taking Dr. Barbara's herbal supplements as directed. These may include liver-supporting herbs such as milk thistle and dandelion root, blood-purifying herbs like burdock root and red clover, and digestive aids such as ginger and peppermint.

- **Dietary Recommendations:** Transition to a clean, whole foods-based diet rich in fruits, vegetables, lean proteins, healthy fats, and fiber. Avoid processed foods, refined sugars, alcohol, and caffeine. Drink plenty of water and herbal teas throughout the day to stay hydrated and support detoxification.

- **Hydration Protocols:** Aim to drink at least eight glasses of water or herbal teas throughout the day to support kidney function and promote the elimination of toxins.

- **Lifestyle Modifications:** Engage in light physical activity such as walking, yoga, or stretching to stimulate circulation and support detoxification. Practice stress-reducing techniques such as deep breathing exercises, meditation, or journaling to promote relaxation and enhance overall well-being.

Days 2-6: Detoxification Phase

- **Herbal Supplements:** Continue taking Dr. Barbara's herbal supplements as directed. These supplements are designed to support detoxification pathways, promote liver and kidney function, and enhance overall cleansing.

- **Dietary Recommendations:** Follow a clean, whole foods-based diet throughout the detoxification phase. Incorporate plenty of leafy greens, cruciferous vegetables, berries, and other antioxidant-rich foods to support detoxification and cellular health. Limit intake of processed foods, refined sugars, and inflammatory foods that may impede detoxification.

- **Hydration Protocols:** Maintain adequate hydration by drinking at least eight glasses of water or herbal teas daily. You may also include hydrating foods such as watermelon, cucumber, and citrus fruits to support hydration and detoxification.

- **Lifestyle Modifications:** Prioritize self-care practices such as gentle exercise, relaxation techniques, and adequate sleep to support detoxification and promote overall well-being. Avoid exposure to environmental toxins, tobacco smoke, and other pollutants that may interfere with detoxification.

Day 7: Transition Phase

- **Herbal Supplements:** Continue taking Dr. Barbara's herbal supplements as directed on the final day of the program.

- **Dietary Recommendations:** Gradually reintroduce solid foods into your diet, starting with easily digestible foods such as soups, steamed vegetables, and lean proteins. Avoid heavy or processed foods that may disrupt digestion or overwhelm detoxification pathways.

- **Hydration Protocols:** Continue to prioritize hydration by drinking plenty of water and herbal teas. You may also include hydrating foods such as fruits and vegetables to support hydration and promote detoxification.

- **Lifestyle Modifications:** Reflect on your experience during the detox program and identify any positive changes or insights gained. Set intentions for maintaining healthy habits moving forward, such as incorporating more whole foods into your diet, practicing stress management techniques, and staying hydrated.

After the 7-Day Program:

- **Maintenance Phase:** Consider incorporating elements of Dr. Barbara's Herbal Detox Protocol into your regular routine to support ongoing detoxification and promote overall health and vitality. This may include taking herbal supplements periodically, following a clean, whole foods-based diet, staying hydrated, and practicing stress-reducing techniques.

- **Follow-Up:** Schedule follow-up appointments with your healthcare provider or a qualified practitioner to assess your progress, address any concerns, and develop a personalized plan for maintaining optimal health and well-being.

In conclusion, Dr. Barbara's Herbal Detox Protocol offers a structured and holistic approach to cleansing the body and rejuvenating health over a seven-day period. By incorporating herbal supplements, dietary recommendations, hydration protocols, and lifestyle modifications, this program supports the body's natural detoxification pathways, promotes organ function, and enhances overall vitality. Whether you're looking to jumpstart a healthier lifestyle, overcome fatigue and digestive issues, or simply rejuvenate your health, Dr. Barbara's Herbal Detox Protocol provides a safe, effective, and transformative solution.

CHAPTER SEVEN

Integrating Alkaline Foods for Enhanced Detoxification

Alkaline foods play a vital role in supporting the body's natural detoxification processes by helping to balance pH levels, reduce inflammation, and promote overall health and vitality. By incorporating alkaline foods into your diet, you can enhance detoxification, support organ function, and optimize cellular health. In this guide, we'll explore the benefits of alkaline foods for detoxification and provide tips for integrating them into your daily meals.

Understanding Alkaline Foods:

Alkaline foods are those that have an alkalizing effect on the body when metabolized, meaning they help raise the pH level of bodily fluids. These foods are typically rich in essential nutrients such as vitamins, minerals, antioxidants, and phytonutrients, which support detoxification and promote overall health. Examples of alkaline foods include fruits, vegetables, leafy greens, nuts, seeds, and certain grains.

Benefits of Alkaline Foods for Detoxification:

1. **Balancing pH Levels:** Alkaline foods help maintain the body's pH balance, which is essential for optimal health. By reducing acidity in the body, alkaline foods support

34

detoxification pathways and promote a more alkaline environment conducive to cellular repair and regeneration.

2. **Reducing Inflammation:** Many alkaline foods have anti-inflammatory properties, which help reduce inflammation and oxidative stress in the body. By lowering inflammation, alkaline foods support detoxification and promote overall well-being.

3. **Supporting Organ Function:** Alkaline foods support the function of organs involved in detoxification, such as the liver, kidneys, and digestive system. By providing essential nutrients and antioxidants, alkaline foods help these organs function optimally and eliminate toxins more efficiently.

4. **Enhancing Cellular Health:** Alkaline foods are rich in antioxidants and phytonutrients that protect cells from damage caused by toxins and free radicals. By nourishing cells and supporting cellular detoxification pathways, alkaline foods promote overall health and vitality.

Tips for Integrating Alkaline Foods into Your Diet:

1. **Emphasize Fruits and Vegetables:** Incorporate a variety of fruits and vegetables into your meals, focusing on alkaline options such as leafy greens, broccoli, cauliflower, cucumber, spinach, kale, avocado, and bell peppers. Aim to

fill half your plate with colorful fruits and vegetables at each meal.

2. **Include Alkaline Proteins:** Choose plant-based protein sources such as legumes, tofu, tempeh, and quinoa, which are alkaline-forming and rich in essential nutrients. These protein sources provide amino acids necessary for cellular repair and support detoxification pathways.

3. **Snack on Nuts and Seeds:** Enjoy nuts and seeds as healthy snacks or add them to salads, smoothies, or oatmeal. Almonds, walnuts, chia seeds, and flaxseeds are excellent sources of healthy fats, fiber, and essential nutrients that support detoxification and promote overall health.

4. **Hydrate with Alkaline Beverages:** Drink plenty of water throughout the day to stay hydrated and support detoxification. You can also enjoy alkaline beverages such as herbal teas, green juices, and coconut water, which help hydrate the body and provide essential nutrients.

5. **Limit Acidic Foods:** Minimize consumption of acidic foods such as processed meats, refined sugars, fried foods, and alcohol, which can disrupt pH balance and hinder detoxification. Instead, focus on alkaline-forming foods that support detoxification and promote overall health.

6. **Experiment with Alkaline Recipes:** Get creative in the kitchen and experiment with alkaline recipes that incorporate a variety of fruits, vegetables, whole grains, and plant-based proteins. Explore different cooking methods such as steaming, roasting, sautéing, and blending to retain the nutrient content of alkaline foods.

Conclusion:

In conclusion, integrating alkaline foods into your diet is an effective way to enhance detoxification, support organ function, and promote overall health and vitality. By emphasizing fruits, vegetables, leafy greens, nuts, seeds, and alkaline proteins, you can nourish your body with essential nutrients and antioxidants that support detoxification pathways and cellular health. Whether enjoyed as part of a balanced meal or incorporated into healthy snacks and beverages, alkaline foods play a crucial role in optimizing health and well-being.

CHAPTER EIGHT

Hydration and Supplements for Optimal Cleansing Results

Hydration and supplementation are integral components of any cleansing or detoxification program, as they support the body's natural detoxification pathways, promote elimination of toxins, and enhance overall well-being. By optimizing hydration and incorporating targeted supplements, you can maximize the effectiveness of your cleansing regimen and achieve optimal results. In this guide, we'll explore the importance of hydration and supplementation for cleansing and provide recommendations for integrating them into your routine.

Hydration for Cleansing:

Hydration plays a crucial role in detoxification, as it helps flush toxins from the body, supports kidney function, and promotes overall cellular health. Adequate hydration ensures that toxins are effectively eliminated through urine, sweat, and respiration, preventing their buildup in tissues and organs. Here are some tips for optimizing hydration during cleansing:

1. **Drink Plenty of Water:** Aim to drink at least 8-10 glasses of water per day, or more if you're engaging in physical activity or sweating heavily. Choose filtered or purified water whenever possible to minimize exposure to contaminants.

2. **Hydrating Foods and Beverages:** Incorporate hydrating foods and beverages into your diet, such as herbal teas, coconut water, water-rich fruits and vegetables (e.g., cucumber, watermelon, oranges), and homemade soups and broths.

3. **Electrolyte Balance:** Maintain electrolyte balance by including foods rich in potassium (e.g., bananas, leafy greens, avocados) and magnesium (e.g., nuts, seeds, dark chocolate) in your diet. You can also supplement with electrolyte powders or tablets to replenish electrolytes lost through sweat and urine.

4. **Monitor Urine Color:** Pay attention to the color of your urine as a hydration indicator. Ideally, urine should be pale yellow in color. Darker urine may indicate dehydration, while clear urine may suggest overhydration.

5. **Hydration Throughout the Day:** Spread out your fluid intake evenly throughout the day rather than consuming large amounts all at once. Sipping water or herbal teas regularly helps maintain hydration levels and supports detoxification.

Supplements for Cleansing:

Supplements can provide targeted support for detoxification pathways, enhance nutrient intake, and promote overall cleansing and vitality. When choosing supplements for cleansing, it's essential to select high-quality products formulated with natural ingredients and backed by scientific research. Here are some supplements commonly used for cleansing:

1. **Liver Support:** Look for supplements containing herbs such as milk thistle, dandelion root, artichoke leaf, and turmeric, which support liver function, enhance bile production, and promote detoxification.

2. **Kidney Support:** Consider supplements containing herbs like nettle leaf, parsley leaf, and juniper berry, which support kidney function, increase urine production, and facilitate toxin elimination.

3. **Digestive Support:** Incorporate digestive enzymes, probiotics, and fiber supplements to support digestive health, enhance nutrient absorption, and promote regular bowel movements. Look for products containing a blend of enzymes (e.g., protease, amylase, lipase), beneficial bacteria (e.g., Lactobacillus, Bifidobacterium), and soluble and insoluble fibers (e.g., psyllium husk, acacia fiber).

4. **Antioxidants:** Include antioxidant supplements such as vitamin C, vitamin E, selenium, and alpha-lipoic acid to neutralize free radicals, reduce oxidative stress, and protect cells from damage during cleansing.

5. **Herbal Detox Blends:** Consider comprehensive herbal detox blends containing a combination of liver-supporting herbs,

blood-purifying herbs, and antioxidant-rich botanicals. These blends are formulated to provide comprehensive support for detoxification and promote overall cleansing and vitality.

Integration into Your Cleansing Protocol:

1. **Consultation with a Healthcare Professional:** Before starting any cleansing or supplementation regimen, consult with a qualified healthcare professional, such as a naturopathic doctor or registered dietitian. They can assess your individual health needs, provide personalized recommendations, and monitor your progress throughout the cleansing process.

2. **Tailored Approach:** Customize your hydration and supplementation protocol based on your unique health goals, dietary preferences, and any underlying health conditions or medications. Adjust fluid intake and supplement dosages as needed to optimize hydration and support detoxification.

3. **Consistency and Compliance:** Maintain consistency with your hydration and supplementation regimen to maximize cleansing results. Follow the recommended dosage instructions for supplements and prioritize hydration throughout the day to support detoxification and overall well-being.

4. **Monitor Progress:** Pay attention to how your body responds to hydration and supplementation during cleansing. Monitor changes in energy levels, digestion, skin health, and overall well-being to assess the effectiveness of your protocol and make adjustments as needed.

By prioritizing hydration and incorporating targeted supplements into your cleansing protocol, you can enhance detoxification, support organ function, and promote overall health and vitality. With a balanced approach and guidance from healthcare professionals, you can achieve optimal cleansing results and embark on a path to improved well-being.

CHAPTER NINE

Addressing Detox Symptoms and Challenges

Embarking on a detoxification journey can be a transformative experience, but it may also come with its share of challenges and symptoms as the body adjusts to cleansing and releasing toxins. Understanding common detox symptoms and knowing how to address them effectively is essential for a successful and enjoyable cleansing process. In this guide, we'll explore various detox symptoms and challenges and provide strategies for managing them to support your well-being throughout your detox journey.

Common Detox Symptoms:

1. **Fatigue:** Feeling tired or lethargic is a common detox symptom as the body expends energy to eliminate toxins and undergoes metabolic changes. Fatigue may be especially pronounced during the initial stages of detoxification.

2. **Headaches:** Headaches or migraines may occur as the body detoxifies and releases toxins, leading to temporary imbalances and increased toxin load in the bloodstream.

3. **Digestive Issues:** Digestive disturbances such as bloating, gas, constipation, or diarrhea may arise as the body adjusts to dietary changes, increased fiber intake, or shifts in gut microbiota during detoxification.

4. **Skin Breakouts:** Skin eruptions, acne flare-ups, or rashes may occur as the body eliminates toxins through the skin, which is one of the body's primary detoxification pathways.

5. **Mood Swings:** Changes in mood, irritability, anxiety, or emotional sensitivity may occur as toxins are released from tissues and organs, impacting neurotransmitter levels and brain function.

Strategies for Addressing Detox Symptoms:

1. **Hydration:** Stay well-hydrated by drinking plenty of water and herbal teas to support the body's detoxification processes, promote toxin elimination, and alleviate detox symptoms such as headaches and fatigue.

2. **Gentle Exercise:** Engage in gentle physical activity such as walking, yoga, or stretching to stimulate circulation, lymphatic drainage, and sweat production, facilitating the elimination of toxins and promoting overall well-being.

3. **Supportive Nutrition:** Focus on nutrient-dense, whole foods that support detoxification and provide essential vitamins, minerals, antioxidants, and fiber. Incorporate plenty of fruits, vegetables, leafy greens, healthy fats, and lean proteins into your diet to nourish your body and alleviate detox symptoms.

4. **Herbal Support:** Consider incorporating herbal supplements or teas that support detoxification and promote organ function, such as milk thistle, dandelion root, ginger, or peppermint. These herbs can help alleviate digestive issues, support liver and kidney function, and enhance overall cleansing.

5. **Stress Management:** Practice stress-reducing techniques such as meditation, deep breathing exercises, mindfulness, or gentle yoga to promote relaxation, reduce cortisol levels, and support overall well-being during detoxification.

6. **Gradual Detoxification:** If detox symptoms are too severe, consider slowing down the detoxification process or gradually introducing dietary and lifestyle changes to allow the body to adjust more comfortably. Listen to your body's signals and adjust your detox protocol as needed to support your well-being.

7. **Professional Guidance:** Seek guidance from qualified healthcare professionals, such as naturopathic doctors, nutritionists, or registered dietitians, who can provide personalized recommendations, monitor your progress, and offer support throughout your detox journey.

Challenges During Detoxification:

1. **Cravings and Withdrawal:** Cravings for unhealthy foods, caffeine, sugar, or other addictive substances may arise

during detoxification, leading to withdrawal symptoms such as headaches, irritability, or mood swings.

2. **Social Pressures:** Social gatherings, events, or peer pressure may present challenges during detoxification, as you navigate dietary restrictions or lifestyle changes while interacting with others.

3. **Herxheimer Reaction:** In some cases, detoxification may lead to a temporary worsening of symptoms known as the Herxheimer reaction, as the body eliminates toxins more rapidly than it can process them. This may manifest as flu-like symptoms, fatigue, or malaise.

Strategies for Overcoming Detox Challenges:

1. **Mindful Eating:** Practice mindful eating and listen to your body's hunger and satiety cues during detoxification. Focus on nourishing foods that support your health goals and provide satisfaction without triggering cravings.

2. **Social Support:** Seek support from friends, family members, or online communities who understand and respect your detox goals. Communicate your needs and boundaries with others to navigate social situations and maintain your commitment to cleansing.

3. **Self-Care Practices:** Prioritize self-care practices such as adequate sleep, relaxation techniques, journaling, or hobbies

that bring you joy and fulfillment during detoxification. Engaging in activities that nourish your mind, body, and spirit can help alleviate stress and promote overall well-being.

4. **Flexibility and Adaptability:** Be flexible and adaptable in your approach to detoxification, recognizing that it's okay to modify your protocol or make adjustments based on your individual needs and circumstances. Listen to your body's signals and honor your intuition as you navigate detox challenges.

5. **Professional Support:** If detox challenges become overwhelming or persist despite your efforts, seek guidance from qualified healthcare professionals who can offer additional support, guidance, or alternative strategies to help you overcome obstacles and achieve your detox goals.

In conclusion, addressing detox symptoms and challenges requires a holistic approach that prioritizes hydration, supportive nutrition, stress management, and self-care practices. By implementing strategies to support your body's natural detoxification processes and navigating challenges with resilience and flexibility, you can experience the transformative benefits of cleansing while promoting overall health and well-being. Remember to listen to your body, honor your needs, and seek support when needed to make your detox journey a positive and empowering experience.

CHAPTER TEN

Maintaining Long-Term Wellness: Post-Detox Lifestyle Strategies

Completing a detoxification program is just the beginning of your wellness journey. To sustain the benefits of cleansing and promote long-term vitality, it's essential to adopt healthy lifestyle habits that support your body's natural detoxification processes and overall well-being. In this guide, we'll explore post-detox lifestyle strategies to help you maintain optimal health and vitality in the long term.

1. Balanced Nutrition:

Transitioning to a balanced and nourishing diet is crucial for maintaining long-term wellness after completing a detox program. Focus on incorporating whole, nutrient-dense foods into your meals, including plenty of fruits, vegetables, lean proteins, healthy fats, and fiber-rich grains. Aim to minimize processed foods, refined sugars, and artificial additives, which can burden the body's detoxification pathways and contribute to inflammation and oxidative stress.

2. Hydration:

Continue prioritizing hydration by drinking plenty of water and herbal teas throughout the day. Proper hydration supports detoxification, promotes optimal organ function, and helps maintain cellular health. Aim to drink at least 8-10 glasses of water daily, adjusting your intake based on activity level, climate, and individual needs.

3. Regular Physical Activity:

Incorporate regular exercise into your daily routine to support overall health and vitality. Engage in a variety of physical activities that you enjoy, such as walking, jogging, cycling, yoga, or strength training. Regular exercise stimulates circulation, promotes lymphatic drainage, and supports detoxification by facilitating the elimination of toxins through sweat and respiration.

4. Stress Management:

Practice stress management techniques to reduce cortisol levels, promote relaxation, and support overall well-being. Incorporate mindfulness practices such as meditation, deep breathing exercises, or progressive muscle relaxation into your daily routine. Prioritize activities that bring you joy and fulfillment, such as spending time in nature, pursuing hobbies, or connecting with loved ones.

5. Quality Sleep:

Prioritize quality sleep to support detoxification, cellular repair, and overall health. Aim for 7-9 hours of restorative sleep each night, establishing a regular sleep schedule and creating a relaxing bedtime routine. Create a sleep-friendly environment by minimizing exposure to electronic devices, caffeine, and stimulating activities before bedtime.

6. Mindful Eating:

Practice mindful eating by paying attention to hunger and satiety cues, savoring each bite, and eating slowly and attentively. Choose whole, minimally processed foods that nourish your body and support your health goals. Be mindful of portion sizes and avoid distractions such as screens or multitasking while eating.

7. Limit Toxin Exposure:

Minimize exposure to environmental toxins by choosing organic, pesticide-free foods whenever possible, using natural cleaning and personal care products, and avoiding exposure to pollutants and toxins in the air and water. Consider incorporating periodic detoxification protocols or cleansing rituals into your routine to support ongoing toxin elimination and promote overall well-being.

8. Continued Learning and Growth:

Stay informed about the latest research and developments in health and wellness to continually refine and enhance your lifestyle habits. Remain open to exploring new strategies, practices, and modalities that support your holistic well-being. Cultivate a growth mindset and embrace opportunities for learning, personal development, and self-discovery.

9. Professional Support:

Seek guidance from qualified healthcare professionals, such as naturopathic doctors, registered dietitians, or holistic practitioners, who can provide personalized recommendations, monitor your progress, and offer support and guidance on your wellness journey. Build a collaborative healthcare team that supports your holistic well-being and addresses your individual health needs.

10. Self-Compassion and Self-Care:

Practice self-compassion and self-care as you navigate your wellness journey. Be gentle with yourself, celebrate your progress, and acknowledge that optimal health is a lifelong journey. Prioritize self-care practices that nurture your physical, mental, and emotional well-being, and make time for activities that bring you joy, fulfillment, and inner peace.

In conclusion, maintaining long-term wellness after completing a detox program requires a holistic approach that prioritizes balanced nutrition, hydration, regular physical activity, stress management, quality sleep, mindful eating, toxin avoidance, continued learning, professional support, and self-compassion. By integrating these post-detox lifestyle strategies into your daily routine, you can sustain the benefits of cleansing, promote optimal health and vitality, and cultivate a lifestyle that supports your holistic well-being for years to come.

BONUS: SOME HERBAL REMEDIES TO KNOW

Cleavers:

Definition: Cleavers, scientifically known as Galium aparine, is a herbaceous annual plant native to Europe, North America, Asia, and Australia. It has a long history of use in traditional medicine for its potential health benefits.

Ingredients: Cleavers contains various bioactive compounds, including iridoid glycosides, flavonoids, tannins, and mucilage. These compounds are believed to contribute to the herb's medicinal properties, including its potential as a diuretic, lymphatic tonic, and mild astringent.

How to Prepare: Cleavers is typically consumed as an herbal tea, infusion, or in fresh salads. To make tea, dried cleavers leaves and stems are steeped in hot water for several minutes before being strained and consumed. It can also be used topically as a poultice or infused oil for skin conditions.

Dosage: The appropriate dosage of cleavers can vary depending on factors such as age, health status, and the specific preparation being used. It's important to follow the recommended dosage on the product label or consult with a qualified herbalist or healthcare professional for personalized guidance.

How to Use: Cleavers tea, infusion, or fresh leaves are typically taken orally. It's often used to support lymphatic drainage, promote urinary tract health, and soothe inflammation. Topically, cleavers can be applied to the skin to alleviate itching, irritation, or minor wounds.

Side Effects: Cleavers is generally considered safe for most people when consumed in moderate amounts. However, some individuals may experience allergic reactions or gastrointestinal upset. It may also interact with certain medications or have adverse effects in individuals with certain health conditions. Pregnant or breastfeeding individuals should consult with a healthcare professional before using cleavers supplements. It's important to use cleavers under the guidance of a healthcare professional and to discontinue use if any adverse effects occur.

Goldenseal:

Definition: Goldenseal, scientifically known as Hydrastis canadensis, is a perennial herb native to North America. It has a long history of use in traditional Native American medicine and later in folk medicine for its potential health benefits.

Ingredients: Goldenseal root contains various bioactive compounds, including alkaloids (such as berberine and hydrastine), flavonoids, and volatile oils. These compounds are believed to contribute to the herb's medicinal properties, including its potential as an antimicrobial, anti-inflammatory, and immune enhancer.

How to Prepare: Goldenseal is typically consumed as an herbal tea, tincture, or in supplement form (such as capsules or tablets). To make tea, dried goldenseal root or leaves are steeped in hot water for several minutes before being strained and consumed.

Dosage: The appropriate dosage of goldenseal can vary depending on factors such as age, health status, and the specific preparation being used. It's important to follow the recommended dosage on the product label or consult with a qualified herbalist or healthcare professional for personalized guidance.

How to Use: Goldenseal tea, tincture, or supplements are typically taken orally. It's often used to support immune function, promote digestive health, and soothe inflammation.

Side Effects: Goldenseal is generally considered safe for most people when used in moderate amounts. However, some individuals may experience mild side effects such as gastrointestinal upset or allergic reactions. It may also interact with certain medications or have adverse effects in individuals with certain health conditions, such as high blood pressure or pregnancy. It's important to use goldenseal under the guidance of a healthcare professional and to discontinue use if any adverse effects occur.

Bio Ferro Tonic:

Definition: Bio Ferro Tonic is a dietary supplement primarily composed of herbs and minerals. It's often marketed as a natural way to support overall health, particularly by promoting blood health and circulation.

Ingredients: Typical ingredients in Bio Ferro Tonic may include a blend of herbs such as burdock root, yellow dock root, sarsaparilla root, and cascara sagrada bark, along with minerals like iron and potassium phosphate.

How to Prepare: Bio Ferro Tonic usually comes in liquid form and is typically taken orally. It's important to follow the instructions on the product label for dosage and administration.

Dosage: The dosage can vary depending on the specific product and individual needs. It's crucial to consult with a healthcare professional or follow the recommended dosage on the product label to avoid potential side effects.

How to Use: Bio Ferro Tonic is often taken by adding the recommended dosage to water or juice and consuming it orally. It's important to shake the bottle well before use and store it according to the manufacturer's instructions.

Side Effects: While Bio Ferro Tonic is generally considered safe when used as directed, some individuals may experience side effects such as digestive discomfort, allergic reactions, or interactions with medications. It's essential to consult with a healthcare provider before starting any new supplement regimen, especially if you have underlying health conditions or are taking medications.

Bladderwrack:

Definition: Bladderwrack is a type of seaweed or marine algae commonly used in traditional medicine and as a dietary supplement. It's known for its potential health benefits, particularly related to thyroid health and weight management.

Ingredients: Bladderwrack contains various nutrients, including iodine, vitamins, minerals, and antioxidants. The primary active components are iodine and fucoidan, a type of carbohydrate found in brown seaweeds.

How to Prepare: Bladderwrack supplements are available in various forms, including capsules, powders, and liquid extracts. They can be taken orally with water or added to smoothies and other beverages.

Dosage: The appropriate dosage of bladderwrack can vary based on factors such as age, health status, and the specific product being used. It's essential to follow the recommended dosage on the product label or consult with a healthcare professional for personalized guidance.

How to Use: Bladderwrack supplements are typically taken orally, either with water or mixed into food or beverages. It's important to follow the instructions on the product label and avoid exceeding the recommended dosage.

Side Effects: While bladderwrack is generally considered safe for most people when used in moderation, excessive intake of iodine from bladderwrack supplements can cause thyroid dysfunction and other adverse effects. Individuals with thyroid disorders, iodine sensitivity, or certain medical conditions should exercise caution and consult with a healthcare provider before using bladderwrack supplements. Common side effects may include digestive upset, allergic reactions, or interactions with medications.

Blood Purifier:

Definition: Blood purifiers are herbal remedies or dietary supplements believed to cleanse or detoxify the blood, often promoting overall health and well-being. They are thought to support the body's natural detoxification processes and improve blood circulation.

Ingredients: Blood purifiers may contain a variety of herbs and botanical extracts known for their purported cleansing and detoxifying properties. Common ingredients include burdock root, red clover, dandelion root, and yellow dock root, among others.

How to Prepare: Blood purifiers are typically available in various forms, including capsules, tablets, powders, and liquid extracts. They are usually taken orally with water or juice, following the recommended dosage on the product label.

Dosage: The dosage of blood purifiers can vary depending on the specific product and individual needs. It's important to adhere to the recommended dosage on the product label or consult with a healthcare professional for personalized guidance.

How to Use: Blood purifiers are typically taken orally, either with water or mixed into beverages. They are often used as part of a detoxification regimen or to support overall health and vitality.

Side Effects: While blood purifiers are generally considered safe for most people when used as directed, some individuals may experience side effects such as digestive discomfort, allergic reactions, or interactions with medications. It's important to consult with a healthcare provider before starting any new supplement regimen, especially if you have underlying health conditions or are taking medications.

Blue Vervain:

Definition: Blue vervain, also known as Verbena hastata, is a perennial herb native to North America. It has been used in traditional medicine for centuries to treat various ailments, including anxiety, insomnia, and digestive issues.

Ingredients: Blue vervain contains several active compounds, including aucubin, verbenalin, and volatile oils. These compounds are believed to contribute to the herb's medicinal properties.

How to Prepare: Blue vervain is typically consumed as a tea or tincture. To make tea, dried blue vervain leaves and flowers are steeped in hot water for several minutes before being strained and consumed. Tinctures are prepared by steeping the herb in alcohol or vinegar to extract its active compounds.

Dosage: The appropriate dosage of blue vervain can vary depending on factors such as age, health status, and the specific preparation being used. It's important to follow the recommended dosage on the product label or consult with a qualified herbalist or healthcare professional for personalized guidance.

How to Use: Blue vervain tea or tincture is typically taken orally. It can be consumed on its own or mixed with honey or other herbal teas for added flavor.

Side Effects: While blue vervain is generally considered safe for most people when used in moderation, excessive intake may cause digestive upset or allergic reactions in some individuals. Pregnant or breastfeeding women should avoid blue vervain due to its potential to stimulate uterine contractions. As with any herbal remedy, it's important to consult with a healthcare provider before using blue vervain, especially if you have underlying health conditions or are taking medications.

Bromide Plus Powder:

Definition: Bromide Plus Powder is a dietary supplement formulated to support thyroid health and promote overall well-being. It typically contains a blend of herbs and minerals that are believed to have beneficial effects on thyroid function.

Ingredients: Bromide Plus Powder often contains a combination of herbs such as bladderwrack, sea moss, and burdock root, along with minerals like iodine and potassium phosphate. These ingredients are thought to support thyroid function and maintain optimal iodine levels in the body.

How to Prepare: Bromide Plus Powder is usually mixed with water or juice to create a drinkable solution. It's important to follow the instructions on the product label for dosage and preparation.

Dosage: The dosage of Bromide Plus Powder can vary depending on the specific product and individual needs. It's crucial to consult with a healthcare professional or follow the recommended dosage on the product label to avoid potential side effects.

How to Use: Bromide Plus Powder is typically taken orally by mixing the recommended dosage with water or juice. It's important to shake or stir the mixture well before consuming it to ensure even distribution of the ingredients.

Side Effects: While Bromide Plus Powder is generally considered safe when used as directed, some individuals may experience side effects such as digestive discomfort or allergic reactions to certain ingredients. It's essential to consult with a healthcare provider before starting any new supplement regimen, especially if you have underlying health conditions or are taking medications.

Bugleweed:

Definition: Bugleweed, also known as Lycopusvirginicus, is a perennial herb native to North America and Europe. It has been used in traditional medicine to treat various conditions, including hyperthyroidism, anxiety, and insomnia.

Ingredients: Bugleweed contains several active compounds, including lithospermic acid, phenolic acids, and flavonoids. These compounds are believed to contribute to the herb's medicinal properties, particularly its ability to regulate thyroid function.

How to Prepare: Bugleweed is commonly consumed as a tea or tincture. To make tea, dried bugleweed leaves and flowers are steeped in hot water for several minutes before being strained and consumed. Tinctures are prepared by steeping the herb in alcohol or vinegar to extract its active compounds.

Dosage: The appropriate dosage of bugleweed can vary depending on factors such as age, health status, and the specific preparation being used. It's important to follow the recommended dosage on the product label or consult with a qualified herbalist or healthcare professional for personalized guidance.

How to Use: Bugleweed tea or tincture is typically taken orally. It can be consumed on its own or mixed with honey or other herbal teas for added flavor.

Side Effects: While bugleweed is generally considered safe for most people when used in moderation, excessive intake may cause digestive upset or allergic reactions in some individuals. Pregnant or breastfeeding women should avoid bugleweed due to its potential to stimulate uterine contractions. As with any herbal remedy, it's important to consult with a healthcare provider before using bugleweed, especially if you have underlying health conditions or are taking medications.

Burdock:

Definition: Burdock, scientifically known as Arctium lappa, is a biennial plant native to Europe and Asia but now found worldwide. It's part of the Asteraceae family and has been used for centuries in traditional medicine and culinary practices.

Ingredients: Burdock contains various nutrients, including carbohydrates, fiber, vitamins (such as vitamin B6, folate, and vitamin C), and minerals (including potassium, magnesium, and manganese). It also contains active compounds such as polyphenols and volatile oils.

How to Prepare: Burdock can be prepared and consumed in various ways. The roots, leaves, and seeds are all utilized for different purposes. The root is commonly used in cooking, herbal teas, tinctures, and supplements, while the leaves and seeds are sometimes used in herbal preparations.

Dosage: The appropriate dosage of burdock root can vary depending on the specific form and intended use. For culinary purposes, there are no strict dosage guidelines, but for supplements or herbal remedies, it's essential to follow the recommended dosage on the product label or consult with a healthcare professional.

How to Use: Burdock root can be used in cooking by peeling, slicing, and adding it to soups, stews, stir-fries, or salads. It can also be brewed into a tea or used to make tinctures or extracts for medicinal purposes. Some people may also take burdock root supplements in capsule or powder form.

Side Effects: While burdock is generally considered safe for most people when consumed in moderate amounts, some individuals may experience allergic reactions or digestive upset. Additionally, burdock may interact with certain medications or have adverse effects in individuals with certain health conditions, such as diabetes or allergies to plants in the Asteraceae family. It's important to consult with a healthcare provider before using burdock, especially if you have underlying health conditions or are taking medications.

Cascara Sagrada:

Definition: Cascara Sagrada, scientifically known as Rhamnus purshiana, is a species of buckthorn native to western North America. It has been used traditionally as a laxative and to promote bowel regularity.

Ingredients: The primary active ingredients in cascara sagrada are anthraquinone glycosides, particularly cascarosides A and B. These compounds stimulate peristalsis in the colon, leading to increased bowel movements.

How to Prepare: Cascara sagrada is typically prepared as an herbal tea, tincture, or capsule. To make tea, dried cascara sagrada bark is steeped in hot water for several minutes before being strained and consumed. Tinctures are prepared by steeping the bark in alcohol to extract its active compounds.

Dosage: The appropriate dosage of cascara sagrada can vary depending on the specific preparation and intended use. It's important to follow the recommended dosage on the product label or consult with a healthcare professional for personalized guidance.

How to Use: Cascara sagrada tea or tincture is typically taken orally. It's important to start with a low dose and gradually increase if needed to avoid potential side effects such as cramping or diarrhea.

Side Effects: Cascara sagrada is considered safe for short-term use when used as directed. However, long-term or excessive use may lead to dependence, electrolyte imbalance, or dehydration. It may also interact with certain medications or have adverse effects in individuals with certain health conditions. It's important to use cascara sagrada under the guidance of a healthcare professional and to discontinue use if any adverse effects occur.

Cell Food:

Definition: Cell Food is a dietary supplement marketed as a highly oxygenating and alkalizing formula. It's claimed to support overall health and vitality by providing essential nutrients and oxygen to the cells.

Ingredients: The exact ingredients of Cell Food can vary depending on the brand, but it typically contains a proprietary blend of minerals, enzymes, electrolytes, and trace elements. Some common ingredients may include purified water, dissolved oxygen, seawater extract, and plant-based enzymes.

How to Prepare: Cell Food is usually available in liquid form and is typically taken orally. It can be consumed directly or diluted in water or juice before consumption.

Dosage: The dosage of Cell Food can vary depending on the specific product and individual needs. It's important to follow the recommended dosage on the product label or consult with a healthcare professional for personalized guidance.

How to Use: Cell Food is typically taken orally, either directly or mixed into water or juice. It's important to shake the bottle well before use and to store it according to the manufacturer's instructions.

Side Effects: Cell Food is generally considered safe for most people when used as directed. However, some individuals may experience mild digestive upset or allergic reactions to certain ingredients. It's essential to consult with a healthcare provider before starting any new supplement regimen, especially if you have underlying health conditions or are taking medications.

Chaparral:

Definition: Chaparral, scientifically known as Larrea tridentata, is a shrub native to the southwestern United States and northern Mexico. It has been used for centuries by Native American tribes for its medicinal properties and is commonly used in herbal medicine today.

Ingredients: Chaparral contains several bioactive compounds, including nordihydroguaiaretic acid (NDGA), flavonoids, lignans, and volatile oils. NDGA is believed to be the primary active compound responsible for many of chaparral's therapeutic effects.

How to Prepare: Chaparral can be prepared and consumed in various forms, including teas, tinctures, capsules, and topical preparations. To make tea, dried chaparral leaves are steeped in hot water for several minutes before being strained and consumed. Tinctures are prepared by steeping the herb in alcohol or vinegar to extract its active compounds.

Dosage: The appropriate dosage of chaparral can vary depending on the specific form and intended use. It's important to follow the recommended dosage on the product label or consult with a healthcare professional for personalized guidance.

How to Use: Chaparral tea or tincture is typically taken orally. It can also be applied topically to the skin for certain conditions. It's important to use chaparral products as directed and to discontinue use if any adverse effects occur.

Side Effects: Chaparral is generally considered safe for most people when used in moderate amounts. However, excessive intake or prolonged use may lead to liver toxicity or other adverse effects. It may also interact with certain medications or have adverse effects in individuals with certain health conditions. It's important to use chaparral under the guidance of a healthcare professional and to discontinue use if any adverse effects occur.

Dandelion Root:

Definition: Dandelion, scientifically known as Taraxacum officinale, is a common flowering plant found worldwide. While often considered a pesky weed, dandelion has a long history of use in traditional medicine for its various health benefits.

Ingredients: Dandelion root contains several bioactive compounds, including sesquiterpene lactones, triterpenes, flavonoids, and polysaccharides. These compounds are believed to contribute to the herb's medicinal properties, including its potential as a diuretic, digestive aid, and liver tonic.

How to Prepare: Dandelion root can be prepared and consumed in various forms, including teas, tinctures, capsules, and extracts. To make tea, dried dandelion root is steeped in hot water for several minutes before being strained and consumed. Tinctures are prepared by steeping the root in alcohol or vinegar to extract its active compounds.

Dosage: The appropriate dosage of dandelion root can vary depending on factors such as age, health status, and the specific preparation being used. It's important to follow the recommended dosage on the product label or consult with a qualified herbalist or healthcare professional for personalized guidance.

How to Use: Dandelion root tea, tincture, or capsules are typically taken orally. It's important to use dandelion root products as directed and to discontinue use if any adverse effects occur.

Side Effects: Dandelion root is generally considered safe for most people when used in moderate amounts. However, some individuals may experience allergic reactions or digestive upset. It may also interact with certain medications or have adverse effects in individuals with certain health conditions. It's important to use dandelion root under the guidance of a healthcare professional and to discontinue use if any adverse effects occur.

Green Food Plus:

Definition: Green Food Plus is a dietary supplement formulated to provide a concentrated source of nutrients derived from various green plants. It's designed to support overall health and well-being by delivering essential vitamins, minerals, antioxidants, and phytonutrients.

Ingredients: Green Food Plus typically contains a blend of powdered green vegetables, grasses, algae, and other plant-based ingredients. Common ingredients may include wheatgrass, barley grass, spirulina, chlorella, alfalfa, kale, spinach, and broccoli, among others.

How to Prepare: Green Food Plus is usually available in powder form and can be mixed with water, juice, or smoothies. It's important to follow the recommended dosage on the product label and to consume it as part of a balanced diet.

Dosage: The appropriate dosage of Green Food Plus can vary depending on the specific product and individual needs. It's important to follow the recommended dosage on the product label or consult with a healthcare professional for personalized guidance.

How to Use: Green Food Plus powder is typically mixed with water, juice, or smoothies and consumed orally. It's often taken once or twice daily, preferably with meals, to maximize nutrient absorption.

Side Effects: Green Food Plus is generally considered safe for most people when used as directed. However, some individuals may experience digestive upset or allergic reactions to certain ingredients. It's important to consult with a healthcare provider before starting any new supplement regimen, especially if you have underlying health conditions or are taking medications.

Guaco:

Definition: Guaco, also known as Mikania cordata or Mikania glomerata, is a medicinal plant native to Central and South

America. It has a long history of use in traditional medicine for its potential therapeutic properties.

Ingredients: Guaco contains several bioactive compounds, including coumarins, flavonoids, tannins, and saponins. These compounds are believed to contribute to the herb's medicinal properties, including its potential as an expectorant, anti-inflammatory, and antispasmodic agent.

How to Prepare: Guaco is typically prepared and consumed as an herbal tea or infusion. To make tea, dried guaco leaves are steeped in hot water for several minutes before being strained and consumed.

Dosage: The appropriate dosage of guaco can vary depending on factors such as age, health status, and the specific preparation being used. It's important to follow the recommended dosage on the product label or consult with a qualified herbalist or healthcare professional for personalized guidance.

How to Use: Guaco tea is typically taken orally. It can be consumed on its own or mixed with honey or other herbal teas for added flavor.

Side Effects: Guaco is generally considered safe for most people when used in moderate amounts. However, some individuals may experience allergic reactions or digestive upset. It may also interact with certain medications or have adverse effects in individuals with certain health conditions. It's important to use guaco under the guidance of a healthcare professional and to discontinue use if any adverse effects occur.

Cocolmeca:

Definition: Cocolmeca, also known as Smilax ornata or sarsaparilla, is a flowering vine native to Mexico and Central America. It has been used traditionally in Mexican and Central American folk medicine for its purported medicinal properties.

Ingredients: Cocolmeca contains various bioactive compounds, including saponins, flavonoids, and plant sterols. These compounds are believed to contribute to the herb's medicinal properties, including its potential as a diuretic, blood purifier, and anti-inflammatory agent.

How to Prepare: Cocolmeca is commonly prepared and consumed as an herbal tea or decoction. To make tea, dried cocolmeca roots or leaves are steeped in hot water for several minutes before being strained and consumed. Decoctions involve boiling the roots or leaves in water to extract their active compounds.

Dosage: The appropriate dosage of cocolmeca can vary depending on factors such as age, health status, and the specific preparation being used. It's important to follow the recommended dosage on the product label or consult with a qualified herbalist or healthcare professional for personalized guidance.

How to Use: Cocolmeca tea or decoction is typically taken orally. It can also be used topically for certain skin conditions. It's important to use cocolmeca products as directed and to discontinue use if any adverse effects occur.

Side Effects: Cocolmeca is generally considered safe for most people when used in moderate amounts. However, excessive intake may lead to digestive upset or other adverse effects. It may also interact with certain medications or have adverse effects in individuals with certain health conditions. It's important to use cocolmeca under the guidance of a healthcare professional and to discontinue use if any adverse effects occur.

Contribo:

Definition: Contribo, also known as Aristolochiatrilobata, is a vine native to the Caribbean and Central America. It has been used traditionally in folk medicine for various purposes, including as a remedy for digestive issues, inflammation, and pain relief.

Ingredients: Contribo contains several bioactive compounds, including aristolochic acids, flavonoids, and alkaloids. These compounds are believed to contribute to the herb's medicinal properties, including its potential as an anti-inflammatory and analgesic agent.

How to Prepare: Contribo is typically prepared and consumed as an herbal tea or decoction. To make tea, dried contribo leaves or stems are steeped in hot water for several minutes before being strained and consumed. Decoctions involve boiling the leaves or stems in water to extract their active compounds.

Dosage: The appropriate dosage of contribo can vary depending on factors such as age, health status, and the specific preparation being used. It's important to follow the recommended dosage on the product label or consult with a qualified herbalist or healthcare professional for personalized guidance.

How to Use: Contribo tea or decoction is typically taken orally. It's important to use contribo products as directed and to discontinue use if any adverse effects occur.

Side Effects: Contribo contains aristolochic acids, which have been associated with serious adverse effects, including kidney damage and cancer. Due to these safety concerns, the use of contribo is highly discouraged, and it's important to avoid products containing aristolochic acids. Individuals should seek alternative remedies for their health needs.

Hops:

Definition: Hops, scientifically known as Humulus lupulus, is a perennial climbing vine native to Europe, Asia, and North America. It is primarily known for its use in brewing beer but has also been used historically in traditional medicine for its potential health benefits.

Ingredients: Hops flowers contain various bioactive compounds, including bitter acids (such as humulone and lupulone), essential oils, flavonoids, and polyphenols. These compounds are believed to contribute to the herb's medicinal properties, including its potential as a sedative, relaxant, and digestive aid.

How to Prepare: Hops is typically consumed as an herbal tea, tincture, or in supplement form (such as capsules or tablets). To make tea, dried hops flowers are steeped in hot water for several minutes before being strained and consumed.

Dosage: The appropriate dosage of hops can vary depending on factors such as age, health status, and the specific preparation being used. It's important to follow the recommended dosage on the product label or consult with a qualified herbalist or healthcare professional for personalized guidance.

How to Use: Hops tea, tincture, or supplements are typically taken orally. It's often used to promote relaxation, relieve anxiety, and support sleep.

Side Effects: Hops is generally considered safe for most people when used in moderate amounts. However, some individuals may experience mild side effects such as drowsiness, gastrointestinal upset, or allergic reactions. It may also interact with certain medications or have adverse effects in individuals with certain health conditions, such as depression or hormone-sensitive conditions. It's important to use hops under the guidance of a healthcare professional and to discontinue use if any adverse effects occur.

Kelp:

Definition: Kelp refers to several species of large brown algae belonging to the Laminariales order. It is commonly found in underwater forests along rocky coastlines around the world. Kelp has been used for centuries in various cultures, particularly in East Asia, for its nutritional and medicinal properties.

Ingredients: Kelp is rich in various nutrients, including iodine, vitamins (such as vitamin K, vitamin C, and B vitamins), minerals (including calcium, magnesium, and potassium), antioxidants, and fiber. These nutrients are believed to contribute to the seaweed's potential health benefits, including its role in thyroid function, bone health, and immune support.

How to Prepare: Kelp is typically consumed dried, powdered, or in supplement form (such as capsules or tablets). It can also be used in cooking, particularly in soups, salads, and stir-fries. Kelp supplements are available in various forms, including powdered extracts, tablets, and liquid extracts.

Dosage: The appropriate dosage of kelp can vary depending on factors such as age, health status, and the specific preparation being used. It's important to follow the recommended dosage on the product label or consult with a qualified healthcare professional for personalized guidance.

How to Use: Kelp supplements are typically taken orally with water. They can be consumed as part of a daily nutritional regimen to support overall health and well-being. Kelp can also be incorporated into recipes as a flavorful and nutritious ingredient.

Side Effects: While kelp is generally considered safe for most people when consumed in moderate amounts, excessive intake of iodine-rich foods or supplements, including kelp, can lead to thyroid dysfunction or iodine toxicity. Some individuals may also be allergic to seaweed and experience allergic reactions. Pregnant or breastfeeding individuals should consult with a healthcare professional before using kelp supplements. It's important to use kelp under the guidance of a healthcare professional and to discontinue use if any adverse effects occur.

Eucalyptus:

Definition: Eucalyptus refers to a genus of flowering trees and shrubs, primarily native to Australia but also found in other parts of the world. Eucalyptus essential oil, extracted from the leaves of certain species, has a long history of use in traditional medicine for its potential health benefits.

Ingredients: Eucalyptus essential oil contains various bioactive compounds, including eucalyptol (cineole), terpenes, and flavonoids. These compounds are believed to contribute to the oil's medicinal properties, including its potential as an expectorant, decongestant, antiseptic, and anti-inflammatory.

How to Prepare: Eucalyptus essential oil can be used in aromatherapy, diffused in the air, or diluted and applied topically to the skin. It can also be added to steam inhalations or chest rubs to help relieve respiratory symptoms.

Dosage: The appropriate dosage of eucalyptus essential oil can vary depending on factors such as age, health status, and the specific application being used. It's important to follow the recommended dosage on the product label or consult with a qualified aromatherapist or healthcare professional for personalized guidance.

How to Use: Eucalyptus essential oil can be used aromatically, topically, or internally, depending on the intended application. It's often used to alleviate respiratory congestion, soothe sore muscles, promote relaxation, and support overall well-being.

Side Effects: Eucalyptus essential oil is generally considered safe for most people when used appropriately. However, it can be toxic if ingested in large amounts and should not be applied directly to the skin without proper dilution. Some individuals may experience allergic reactions or respiratory irritation when exposed to eucalyptus oil. It's important to use eucalyptus oil with caution, especially around children and pets. Pregnant or breastfeeding individuals should consult with a healthcare professional before using eucalyptus oil. If any adverse effects occur, discontinue use and seek medical attention.

Feverfew:

Definition: Feverfew, scientifically known as Tanacetum parthenium, is a perennial herb native to Europe but also found in other parts of the world. It has a long history of use in traditional medicine, particularly in European folk medicine, for its potential health benefits.

Ingredients: Feverfew contains various bioactive compounds, including sesquiterpene lactones (such as parthenolide), flavonoids, and volatile oils. These compounds are believed to contribute to the herb's medicinal properties, including its potential as an anti-inflammatory, analgesic, and migraine prophylactic.

How to Prepare: Feverfew is typically consumed as an herbal tea, tincture, or in supplement form (such as capsules or tablets). To make tea, dried feverfew leaves and flowers are steeped in hot water for several minutes before being strained and consumed.

Dosage: The appropriate dosage of feverfew can vary depending on factors such as age, health status, and the specific preparation being used. It's important to follow the recommended dosage on the product label or consult with a qualified herbalist or healthcare professional for personalized guidance.

How to Use: Feverfew tea, tincture, or supplements are typically taken orally. It's often used to alleviate headaches, including migraines, and to support overall well-being.

Side Effects: Feverfew is generally considered safe for most people when used in moderate amounts. However, some individuals may experience mild side effects such as gastrointestinal upset or allergic reactions. It may also interact with certain medications or have adverse effects in individuals with certain health conditions, such as bleeding disorders or pregnancy. It's important to use feverfew under the guidance of a healthcare professional and to discontinue use if any adverse effects occur.

Ginseng:

Definition: Ginseng refers to several species of perennial plants belonging to the Panax genus, including Panax ginseng (Asian ginseng) and Panax quinquefolius (American ginseng). Ginseng has been used for centuries in traditional medicine, particularly in East Asia, for its potential health benefits.

Ingredients: Ginseng root contains various bioactive compounds, including ginsenosides, polysaccharides, and peptides. These compounds are believed to contribute to the herb's medicinal properties, including its potential as an adaptogen, immune enhancer, and cognitive booster.

How to Prepare: Ginseng is typically consumed as a powdered root, herbal tea, tincture, or in supplement form (such as capsules or tablets). To make tea, dried ginseng root slices are simmered in water for several minutes before being strained and consumed.

Dosage: The appropriate dosage of ginseng can vary depending on factors such as age, health status, and the specific preparation being used. It's important to follow the recommended dosage on the product label or consult with a qualified herbalist or healthcare professional for personalized guidance.

How to Use: Ginseng powder, tea, tincture, or supplements are typically taken orally. It's often used to support energy levels, enhance cognitive function, and promote overall well-being.

Side Effects: Ginseng is generally considered safe for most people when used in moderate amounts. However, some individuals may experience mild side effects such as insomnia, gastrointestinal upset, or headaches. It may also interact with certain medications or have adverse effects in individuals with certain health conditions, such as high blood pressure or diabetes. Pregnant or breastfeeding individuals should consult with a healthcare professional before using ginseng supplements. It's important to use ginseng under the guidance of a healthcare professional and to discontinue use if any adverse effects occur.

THE END